IBS Cookbook

Irritable Bowel Syndrome Natural Relief
Guide and Cookbook

Charles Seaton

Table of Contents

Chapter 1 – What IBS is all about

Chapter 2 – Causes & Symptoms

Chapter 3 – Food Allergens

Chapter 4 – How Dietary Adjustment Works

Chapter 5 – Recipes for Relief

Chapter 6 – Conclusion

Chapter 1 - What IBS is all about

IBS stands for irritable bowel syndrome. It is a condition characterized by bowel hypersensitivity. The definite cause remains unknown. There is also no definite cure. The symptoms also vary among individuals, and the triggers vary as well. Treatment is mainly through dietary and lifestyle changes.

What happens in IBS

Irritable bowel syndrome is a common disorder of the digestive system that affects that system's function. All parts of the digestive tract are normal and intact when studied closely under a microscope, but the functioning becomes abnormal depending on several factors.

Occurrence

Anybody can be affected by IBS regardless of age and sex. However, statistics show that IBS starts to develop in teenagers and young adults, and persists towards adulthood. Also, it is twice more common among women than among men. The ratio increases to 3:1 in older populations.

Most people seeking medical treatment and who have been diagnosed with IBS for the first time are between the ages 30 and 50 years old. Incidence declines in older populations, specifically people more than 60 years of age.

About 10% to 15% of the population is affected by IBS. But some experts maintain that the numbers may actually be higher, because only a few seek medical attention and some are misdiagnosed with other diseases that have the same symptoms as IBS (sensitivity disorders, celiac, etc.). Its vague symptoms that vary in severity and characteristic among individuals also contribute to misdiagnosis. The symptoms wax and wane over time, and the pattern may sometimes be lost on the person suffering from IBS, lulled into thinking the discomforts are related to some other reason. .

Diagnosis

Diagnosis is mainly recognition and monitoring of symptoms. The symptoms should occur for a total of at least 12 weeks within the last 12 months. The incidence need not be a consecutive 12-week period, as long as the cumulative days that the symptoms were present are 12 weeks. The main symptom to watch out for is pain or discomfort over the abdomen with any 2 of the following features:

- Onset of pain or discomfort is associated with change in the frequency of stool
- Onset of pain or discomfort is associated with change in the appearance, consistency or form of the stool
- Pain and discomfort is relieved with passing stool

The above symptoms should be accompanied by supporting ones such as any of the following:

- Less than 3 bowel movements per week
- More than 3 bowel movements per day
- Stools that are hard and lumpy
- Stools that are loose or have a watery consistency
- Feelings of urgency
- Feelings of incomplete bowel emptying after defecation
- Mucus in the stool
- Bloating and feelings of abdominal fullness

Stool characteristics are also important in diagnosing IBS. If the following are not observed, then there is not enough to consider an IBS diagnosis. IBS associated with constipation:

For at least 12 weeks (not necessarily in consecutive days) in the last 12 months, any 2 of the following should be present. More than 25% of bowel movements show the following:

- Requiring straining
- Yielding hard or lumpy stools
- Ends with feelings of incomplete emptying of the bowels
- Feelings of blockage in the anus
- Needs manual methods to facilitate stool evacuation (e.g., removal of stool by manually inserting the fingers)
- Less than 3 bowel movements a week

Chapter 2 - Symptoms & Risk Factors

The cause of IBS remains unknown, though, through observation, isveral factors have been linked to its development and occurrence. The symptoms also widely vary, from simple stomach discomfort to excruciating pain.

Symptoms

Pain and discomfort are the most common symptoms related to IBS. However, it does not mean that these symptoms automatically lead to a diagnosis. Pain often comes and goes (intermittent). The duration varies greatly. Some describe it as colicky type of pain or spasmic. It may be relieved when passing the stool or gas. The severity also varies from mild discomfort to severe pain.

Some reports bloated feelings, with or without noticeable swelling of the abdomen. It may be accompanied by frequent passing of gas.

Passing of stool also vary from person to person and at each IBS occurrence in the same person. Sometimes, IBS will be accompanied by diarrhea, sometimes constipation. In some, diarrheal episodes alternate with constipation episodes.

Stools can become watery or pass out as ribbons. Sometimes these become small, hard and resemble pellets. Sometimes, mucus accompanies stool.

People affected with IBS sometimes report of feeling incomplete emptying after passing stools. They feel as if they still need to defecate, but sitting on the toilet yields no stool.

Some report feelings of urgency. This is characterized by feelings of needing to go to the toilet quickly. This often happens in the morning, called morning rush. Feelings of urgency happen upon getting up, before or after having breakfast.

Others report digestive problems like:

- Nausea
- Belching
- Poor appetite (anorexia)
- Feels full shortly after eating, despite eating small amounts
- Heart burn

Symptoms may also be unrelated to the digestive functioning, such as:

- Headache
- Backache
- Tiredness
- Generalized muscle pains

Risk Factors

Age

Most IBS diagnoses (about 50%) are made among people in their late 20s to mid 30s.

Sex

Women are at higher risk to develop IBS than men.

Family history

People with 1st degree relative who suffer from IBS have been shown to be at an increased risk for developing IBS.

History of abuse

Studies have shown that people who had a history of abuse are at an increased risk for developing gastrointestinal problems, including IBS.

Triggers

Stress

People suffering from IBS find that their symptoms appear 0r worsen in times of stress. It does not, however, cause IBS. Stressful situations only trigger or aggravate an already existing IBS symptom.

Hormones

Hormonal changes in women occur more often. Women who suffer from IBS report that their symptoms worsen during their menstrual cycle. This association is often considered as an explanation for why more of IBS sufferers are women.

Foods

This is probably the most remarkable of all IBS triggers. People find that eating certain foods worsen symptoms of IBS. Note that foods only worsen symptoms, not cause IBS. Chocolate, alcohol and caffeine have been reported to worsen diarrhea and constipation in IBS sufferers.

Carbonated drinks and fibers in fruits and vegetables are linked to feelings of abdominal discomfort and bloating.

However, while dairy caffeine and artificial sweeteners are also linked to IBS, profound abdominal problems after consumption of these are more related to sugar or lactose sensitivity rather than IBS.

Chapter 3 - Food Allergens

Certain foods have been found to trigger IBS, and food is one of the major trigger or treatment. Foods that commonly trigger IBS symptoms include the following:

Greasy Food

High fat content of greasy foods irritate the digestive tract. It causes intestinal contraction to increase in intensity (strength) and frequency. The body is naturally able to tolerate fats in the diet, even in large amounts. However, in IBS, the body is extra sensitive to the fats. The digestive tract increases its movements to try to remove the fats faster. This results in cramps, pain and diarrhea.

Dairy products

As mentioned earlier, digestive problems from dairy products are more related to lactose intolerance. However, a small number of IBS sufferers do have their symptoms triggered by the lactose found in dairy products.

Lactose coats the lining of the intestines. In IBS, it is often viewed as an irritating substance. The body tries to get rid of it by, again, increasing the digestive tract's wave-like movements to propel the lactose out for excretion. Cramps, bloating and diarrhea results.

Whole grains

Adding food sources high in fiber is important for a healthy and balanced meal. However, fier rich foods also contain the protein gluten. This protein can cause irritation in the lining of the digestive tract. In gluten sensitivity conditions like celiac disease, the immune system recognizes gluten as a foreign substance and attacks it. In IBS, gluten is seen as a tough protein to digest. The longer it stays undigested, the more irritating it becomes to the gut lining. The response is to try to move it out instead of trying or try to digest it faster. Trying to move it out faster results in cramping and diarrhea. Trying to digest it faster results in bloating (as gluten remains undigested), cramps (from too much enzymatic and churning gut movement for digestion), and constipation (as the body tries to retain gluten for further digestion) or diarrhea (effect of greater gut movement).

Whole grain foods mean that the bran of the grain remains intact and is eaten. Bran is a gut irritant because it is difficult to digest.

Whole grain foods are also high in insoluble fiber. This type of fiber remains intact despite the presence of digestive enzymes. As such, the sensitive IBS-affected gut recognizes this undigested compound to be an irritant. The same reaction occurs. The gut tries to eliminate it rapidly while trying to increase the effort in digestion.

Raw fruits

Raw fruits contain an abundance of essential nutrients, minerals, vitamins, phytochemicals and antioxidants. However, some fruits contain irritating compounds that trigger IBS. Citrus fruits like tangerines and oranges are high vitamin C, an acid. Fruits like melons are also rich in fibers and liquids that can be irritating to the lining of the gut. These irritate the gut lining, triggering a response that elicits IBS symptoms.

Some fruits have especially high fructose levels. This compound also irritates the lining of the intestines, triggering IBS symptoms.

Vegetables

While essential in a healthy and balanced diet, some vegetables trigger IBS symptoms. Raw vegetables like peppers, onions and scallions contain powerful compounds that irritate the lining of the gut, compounds like allicin and capsaicin.

Cruciferous vegetables like cabbage and broccoli promote gas production within the digestive tract. Gas promotes bloating and abdominal discomfort, which are also symptoms of IBS.

The above mentioned vegetables are also rich in sulfur. In itself, sulfur compounds are highly irritating in the digestive tract. They also contribute to gas production, which worsen bloating and cramps.

Artificial Sweeteners

Some people have poor tolerance of the chemicals in artificial sweeteners such as aspartame. Artificial sweeteners are used in most sugar-free and diet products. Poor tolerance leads to gas formation within the gut and bloating.

Drinks

Several beverages also trigger or worsen IBS symptoms because of the different chemical compounds they contain. Sodas and carbonated drinks worsen bloating and gas. The carbon gas in these drinks are released once inside the digestive tract and adds to the buildup of gas within the abdomen.

Coffee and caffeinated drinks worsen IBS because of the caffeine content. Caffeine is a digestive stimulant. Drinking beverages that contain this compound will result in worsening the cramps and diarrhea because the intestines are stimulated to move at a more rapid pace.

Alcohol is also a digestive stimulant and irritant. Drinking alcoholic beverages will worsen the already irritated bowel.

Diet sodas and other beverages contain artificial sweeteners, which are poorly tolerated by the body.

Spicy foods

Studies have shown a link between spicy foods and abdominal pain in IBS. It has been found that IBS sufferers have more sensitive nerve endings in the intestines that readily interact with the compounds in spicy foods, particularly chili peppers. Capsaicin compounds in chili, when it reacts with the intestinal nerve endings, produce pain.

Seeds and nuts

Nuts are a problem to people who suffer from IBS because of the high fat content. Other than that, there is no evidence yet of how and why seeds and nuts produce painful flare ups in IBS.

Chocolate

Chocolate can trigger IBS in a number of ways depending on preparation, concentration of cacao and added ingredients. Milk chocolate contains milk, lactose that irritates the intestinal lining. It also contains caffeine, which is a known digestive irritant and stimulant. Other innate chemicals in chocolate may also be irritating, or the body is just unable to tolerate the compounds.

Chapter 4 - IBS FODMAPS

FODMAP means fermentable Oligo-, Di- and Monosaccharides and Polyols. This group of foods contain carbohydrates that have been found to trigger and worsen symptoms related to some digestive disorders like irritable bowel syndrome (IBS) and inflammatory bowel disease (IBD).

Oligosaccharides are carbohydrate forms composed of galactans and fructans. Disaccharides refer to lactose and monosaccharide refers to fructose. Polyols are sugar alcohols such as mannitol, maltitol, xylitol and sorbitol. All these are not easily digested by the body. They also undergo fermentation process the longer they stay within the digestive tract. Fermentation will lead to gas formation and the by-products that are released irritate the gut lining. The entire process contributes to cramps, bloating, constipation and diarrhea that are related to IBS symptoms.

High FODMAP

These foods are to be avoided or at least reduce consumption to a minimum.

Onions and garlic are to be avoided entirely. If not possible, opt to use garlic or onion flavored oils. The irritating compounds are removed in these infused oils. Other foods that are high FODMAP are as follows:

Vegetables

(for their high fiber content and some, for the gas-producing effect)
Asparagus
Artichokes
Beans: baked, kidney, soy, black-eyed, broad, butter
Beet root
Broccoli
Brussels sprouts
Cauliflower
Cabbage
Fennel
Chick peas
Lentils
Green bell peppers
Leeks
Spring onions (white portion)
Scallions
Shallots
Peas
Okra
Mushrooms

Fruits

Avocado – for its high fat and fiber content
For their high fructose contents:
Apricots
Apples
Cherries
Blackberries
Lychee
Pears

Peaches
Nectarines
Prunes
Plums
Watermelon
Cantaloupe

Food made from grain and grain products (like flour)

All products made from wheat such as gravies, sauces and other similar condiments- read labels carefully
Cakes
Breads
Breadcrumbs
Biscuits
Pasta
Noodles
Pastries
Wheat rolls and wheat bread
Wheat cereals
Bran cereals
Rye
Semolina
Couscous
Udon noodles

Nuts

Pistachios

Sweets and Sweeteners

Any sweets labeled as sugar-free- more likely contains artificial sweeteners
Agave
Honey
Fructose- found in a lot of commercially manufactured products
High fructose corn syrup – also found in several commercial food products
Inulin
Mannitol
Isomalt
Xylitol

Sorbitol
Milk chocolate

Prebiotic foods

These are added to foods to improve its nutritional content. However, some of these are irritating to an IBS-affected gut. They are commonly added to yogurt, snack bars and other "healthy" snacks. These are labeled as:

Inulin
Oligofructose
FOS or fructooligosaccharides

Drinks

Certain compound sin drinks are irritating to the gut lining, triggering IBS flare-ups.
Beer- malt and alcohol, plus a few of the fibers can irritate the lining of the intestines, especially in large amounts (more than 1 bottle at a time)
Dandelion tea- plant compounds that have herbal benefits but may irritate the lining of the bowels
Fruit and herbal teas with apple as additive – lignin from apple is an irritant
Orange juice in amounts more than 100 ml at a time- highly acidic and irritating to the gut lining
Fizzy drinks that are sugar free- carbon from the fizz adds to gas in the gut. Sugar-free means use of poorly tolerated artificial sweeteners.
Sports drinks – additives and special formulations are poorly tolerated by the IBS-affected gut
Rum – too much alcohol concentration
Wine – if more than 1 glass

Dairy foods

From lactose, fat and sugar contents
Custard
Margarine
Ice cream
Milk from cow, sheep and goat
Soft cheese like mascarpone, cottage cheese and ricotta
Cheeses with added sugars

All kinds of yogurt, including Greek yogurt

Cooking ingredients

Cocoa powder - concentrated compounds
Extra vegetable oils

Low FODMAP

These foods are good to eat, contain less irritating compounds and are generally well tolerated.

Vegetables

Bean sprouts
Bok choy
Carrots
Butternut squash
Celery
Courgette
Chives
Eggplant
Cucumber
Lettuce
Ginger
Green beans
Red bell peppers
Parsnip
Olives
Parsley
Potato
Spring onions (green part)
Sweet potato
Spinach
Pumpkin
Zucchini
Tomato except cherry tomato

Fish and Seafood
Cod
Haddock
Salmon
Canned tuna
Trout
Plaice
Crab
Lobster
Oysters
Mussels

Shrimp

Fruits

Some fruits have low fructose contents and are generally well tolerated such as:
Boysenberry
Blueberries
Bananas
Clementine
Cranberry
Honeydew melons
Galia melons
Kiwi
Grapefruit
Grape
Dates
Lime
Mandarin oranges (less acidic)
Lemon
Passion fruits
Raisins
Raspberry
Pineapple
Papaya
Strawberry

Some grains and grain products
Wheat-free or gluten free breads
Bread and other baked products made from corn flour, rice flour, barley, potato flour and oats
Pasta- wheat free and gluten free
Rice noodles
Corn flakes
Rice bran
Porridge
Oat-based cereals
Buckwheat noodles
Rice krispies
Barley
Amaranth
Buckwheat

Crisp bread
Corn cakes
Oats
Oatcakes
Millet
Polenta
Rice cakes and rice crackers
Sorghum

Nuts and seeds

Coconut including the cream, milk and flesh

Peanuts – not more than 15 pieces

Macadamia – not more than 10 pieces

Pine nuts – not more than 15 pieces

Pecans – not more than 15 pieces

Walnuts – not more than 10 pieces

Pumpkin seeds – not more than 2 tablespoons

Quinoa

Sunflower seeds – not more than 2 tablespoons

Sesame seeds – not more than 2 tablespoon

Sweets and Sweeteners
IBS sufferers can still enjoy sweets by using any of the following:
Golden syrup
Maple syrup
Sucralose
Saccharine
Glucose

Drinks
Fruits and herbal teas without any apple flavors
Lemonade in small amounts
Water

Dairy Products

Not all dairy products are created equal. Some are low FODMAP and IBS-friendly.
Camembert cheese
Brie cheese
Feta cheese
Parmesan cheese
Swiss cheese
Mozzarella cheese
Dairy-free chocolate pudding
Gelato
Sorbet
Rice milk
Oat milk
Tofu

Chapter 5 - Recipes for Relief

Black Pepper & Kale Chips

Bacon Wrapped Brussels Sprouts

Pancetta Wrapped Shrimp Snacks

Plantain Fries

Baked Cauliflower

Broccoli Fries

Lean Mean Collard Greens

Strawberry Creamy Blast

Baked Sweet Plantains

Grilled Pineapple Fruit Salad

Piña Colada Smoothie

Bacon Mofongo

Smoked Salmon and Avocado Snacks

Garlic Mashed Parsnips

Blueberry Morning Drink

Nutritional Blend

Homemade Applesauce

Bacon and Sweet Potato Hash

Tuna Spread

Olive Tapenade

Quick Raw Avocado Slaw

Parchment Baked Salmon

Peppercorn Crusted Filet Mignon

Seafood Paella

Garlic and Herb Escargot

Chicken and "Rice"

Bacon Baked Apples

Sautéed Mongolian Beef

Southern Liver and Onions

Chicken Garlic Roast

Salmon with Berry Chutney

Holiday Baked Ham

Rack of Lamb with Mint Sauce

Bacon Wrapped Filet Mignon

Herb Roasted Pork Tenderloin

Pan Seared Duck

Apple Venison Roast

Kelp Noodle Chicken Soup

Butternut Squash Soup

New England Clam Chowder

Spinach Artichoke Soup

Cream of Mushroom Soup

Smoked Salmon Avocado Salad

Avocado Persimmon Salad

Kelp Noodle Salad

Salmon & Veggie Breakfast Salad

Black Pepper & Kale Chips

Prep time: 15 minutes

Cook time: 10-15 minutes

INGREDIENTS

1 handful baby kale greens

¼ tsp garlic powder

2 tbsp coconut oil

¼ tsp Celtic sea salt

¼ tsp ground black pepper

INSTRUCTIONS

1. Preheat oven to 350 degrees.
2. In a large bowl, combine 2 tbsp melted coconut oil with kale greens, garlic powder, Celtic sea salt and ground black pepper. Mix well.
3. Line a baking sheet with parchment paper and place kale on it. Bake until the edges of the kale are browned, 10-15 minutes.
4. Remove from oven and cool. Serve.

Bacon Wrapped Brussels Sprouts

Prep Time: 10 minutes

Cook Time: 20 minutes

Servings: 4

INGREDIENTS

24 Brussels sprouts

8 strips nitrate-free bacon

24 wooden toothpicks

1/4 teaspoon ground black pepper

INSTRUCTIONS

1. Preheat oven to 375 degrees F. Place oven-safe wire rack in sheet pan.
2. Soak toothpicks in water for about 5 minutes.
3. Cut bacon strips into thirds. Wrap each Brussels sprout in bacon and use toothpicks to secure.
4. Place bacon wrapped Brussels sprouts on wire rack and sprinkle with pepper.
5. Bake for about 15 - 20 minutes, until bacon is crisp and veggies are cooked through. Remove and let cool about 2 minutes.
6. Serve warm or room temperature.

Pancetta Wrapped Shrimp Snacks

Prep Time: 10 minutes

Cook Time: 15 minutes

Servings: 2

INGREDIENTS

12 jumbo shrimp

4 slices nitrate-free pancetta

12 wooden toothpicks

Ground white pepper, to taste

Celtic sea salt, to taste

INSTRUCTIONS

1. Soak toothpicks in water about 5 minutes.
2. Preheat oven to 350 degrees F. Place oven-safe wire rack in sheet pan.
3. Peel and devein shrimp, leaving tail on. Sprinkle with salt and pepper, to taste.
4. Cut pancetta into thirds. Wrap shrimp in pancetta and secure with toothpick.
5. Place wrapped shrimp on wire rack. Bake for about 15 minutes, or until bacon is crisp and shrimp is just cooked through/ Do not overcook.
6. Remove from oven and transfer to serving dish.

7. Serve hot.

Plantain Fries

Prep Time: 10 minutes

Cook Time: 15

Servings: 1

INGREDIENTS

1 large green plantain

Celtic sea salt, to taste

Ground black pepper, to taste

1/2 lime (optional)

coconut oil (for cooking)

INSTRUCTIONS

1. Bring pot of salted water to boil over medium heat. Heat large pan over medium-high heat. Coat with coconut oil.
2. Cut off ends of plantain. Carefully cut through peel down length of plantain on 4 sides. Remove thick peel.
3. Cut plantain on sharp diagonal to make long angled 1/4 inch slices. Add to boiling water. Cook about 5 minutes, until tender but not mushy.
4. Drain plantains on paper towels and pat to dry. Slice plantains into strips.

5. Add par cooked plantain strips to hot oil. Cook about 2 - 4 minutes on each side, until golden brown and cooked through. Turn with tongs or slotted spoon half way through cooking.

6. Remove cooked plantain from pan and drain on clean paper towels. Transfer to serving dish.

7. Sprinkle with salt and pepper, to taste. Cut lime into wedges and squeeze over dish (optional).

8. Serve hot with lime wedges.

Baked Cauliflower

Prep time:

Cook time:

INGREDIENTS

1 head of cauliflower

3 tbsp extra virgin olive oil

¼ tsp Celtic sea salt

INSTRUCTIONS

1. Preheat oven to 425 degrees.
2. Cut the head of cauliflower down to smaller florets, about an inch or so in length.
3. In a large bowl, combine cauliflower, extra virgin olive oil and Celtic sea salt and mix.
4. Place the cauliflower on a baking sheet and roast for 1 hour. Turn the pieces 4 times during baking at 15 minute intervals.
5. Remove from oven and let cool. Serve.

Broccoli Fries

Prep time: 15 minutes

Cook time: 20 minutes

INGREDIENTS

1 large bunch of broccoli

2 tbsp extra virgin olive oil

1 tbsp garlic powder

¼ tsp Celtic sea salt

INSTRUCTIONS

1. Preheat oven to 450 degrees. Cut the broccoli into florets.
2. In a large bowl, mix broccoli florets, extra virgin olive oil, garlic powder and Celtic sea salt.
3. Spread the broccoli over a baking sheet and roast for 20 minutes until the edges are crispy.
4. Remove from oven and let cool. Serve.

Lean Mean Collard Greens

Prep Time: 15 minutes

Cook Time: 2 1/2 hours

Servings: 8

INGREDIENTS

2 heads (or 2 large bags) fresh collard greens

6 slices nitrate-free bacon (or 1 small ham hock)

8 cups chicken stock

Water

INSTRUCTIONS

1. Preheat oven to 350 degrees F. Heat large pot over medium-high heat.
2. Rinse collards well and roughly chop. Place in large colander or in clean sink to drain.
3. Add bacon or ham hock to hot pot and render down for about 5 minutes.
4. Add greens to pot in batches. If all greens to not fit, reserve. Add chicken stock.
5. Bring pot to a simmer then reduce to low heat. Add any remaining greens, plus enough water just to cover, if necessary. Stir gently.
6. Simmer until collards are tender, about 2 - 2 1/2 hours.
7. Drain greens well. Transfer to serving dish and serve warm.

Strawberry Creamy Blast

Prep time: 3 minutes

INGREDIENTS

3 oz tuna

½ avocado

¼ tsp ground black pepper

½ cup blueberries

½ cup strawberries

INSTRUCTIONS

1. Mix tuna and avocado into a paste. Add ground black pepper and combine.
2. Chop strawberries and add them into blueberries.
3. Place both tuna and fruit mixtures on a plate and serve.

Baked Sweet Plantains

Prep Time: 5 minutes

Cook Time: 20 minutes

Servings: 1

INGREDIENTS

1 ripe yellow plantain

1 tablespoon sweetener*

2 tablespoons water

1 teaspoon coconut oil

1/2 teaspoon ground cinnamon

INSTRUCTIONS

1. Preheat oven to 400 degrees F. Line baking pan with parchment, or lightly coat with coconut oil.
2. Cut plantain into 3/4 inch slices. Remove peel from each slice.
3. Toss plantains in small bowl with sweetener, water, oil and cinnamon.
4. Arrange plantains in single layer on baking pan. Bake 10 minutes, then turn over and bake another 10 minutes, or until plantains are golden brown and tender.
5. Serve warm.

raw honey or agave nectar

Grilled Pineapple Fruit Salad

Prep Time: 5 minutes

Cook Time: 10 minutes

Servings: 4

INGREDIENTS

1/2 pineapple

1 peach

1 cup fresh cherries

1 orange

1 tablespoon fresh mint leaves

Half lemon

INSTRUCTIONS

1. Heat griddle or grill over medium-high heat. Lightly coat with coconut oil.

2. Peel and core pineapple. Cut into half inch slices. Place slice on griddle and grill about 4 - 5 minutes on each side, until grill marks appear and sugars caramelized.

3. Cut peach in half and grill flesh side down for about 5 minutes.

4. Pit cherries and slice in half. Peel orange and cut flesh from white cellulose film and pith.

5. Chop pineapple and peach. Add to medium mixing bowl with cherries and orange wedges. Chiffon mint. Add to bowl and squeeze on lemon juice. Toss to combine.

6. Serve room temperature. Or refrigerate and serve chilled.

Piña Colada Smoothie

Prep Time: 5 minutes

Cook Time: 5 minutes

Servings: 2

INSTRUCTIONS

1 large banana

1 cup pineapple chunks (fresh, frozen or canned)

2 tablespoons flaked coconut

1 cup coconut milk

1 cup ice (crushed preferably)

DIRECTIONS

1. Add banana, pineapple, coconut, coconut milk and ice to highs-speed blender. Process until smooth.
2. Pour into chilled glasses and serve immediately.

Bacon Mofongo

Prep Time: 15 minutes

Cook Time: 15 minutes

Servings: 2

INGREDIENTS

1 green plantain

2 slices nitrate-free bacon

3 garlic cloves

1/4 teaspoon ground black pepper

Bacon drippings

Coconut oil (for cooking)

INSTRUCTIONS

1. Bring medium pot of lightly salted water to boil.

2. Cut plantains into 1 inch slices. Remove peel and add to boiling water. Boil plantains for about 10 minutes, until soft.

3. Heat small pot over medium heat. Dice bacon and add to pot. Sauté and render out fat for about 5 minutes, until bacon is crisp. Pour bacon and drippings into medium bowl to cool slightly.

4. Add 1 inch worth of coconut oil to hot pot.

5. Add slightly cooled bacon and drippings to food processor or bullet blender with peeled garlic. Process until well blended. Add back to medium bowl. Drain plantains and add to bowl with black pepper.

6. Mash plantains and seasonings in bowl with fork or potato masher. Roll mixture into 6 small balls.

7. Carefully add plantain balls to hot oil and fry for about 2 minutes. Turn with tongs half way through cooking. Remove and drain on paper towel.

8. Serve hot.

NOTE: For *Baked Mofongo*, preheat oven to 400 degrees F and bake plantain balls on oiled or parchment covered sheet pan for about 10 minutes, until golden brown.

Smoked Salmon and Avocado Snacks

Prep Time: 5* minutes

Servings: 2

INGREDIENTS

4 oz (1 or 1/2 package) cold-smoked salmon

1 avocado

1 stalk fresh dill

Pinch sea salt

1/2 lemon (optional)

INSTRUCTIONS

1. Slice avocado in half and remove pit. Cut into thick slices in peel then scoop out with large spoon.

2. Slice smoked salmon into long 1 inch strips. Wrap 1 salmon strips around each avocado slice. Arrange wrapped avocado on serving dish.

3. Mince fresh dill. Sprinkle dill and salt over avocado wraps and serve immediately.

4. Or squeeze juice of 1/2 lemon over avocado wraps, sprinkle on dill and salt, and refrigerate 20 minutes. Then serve chilled.

Garlic Mashed Parsnips

Prep Time: 10 minutes

Cook Time: 20 minutes

Servings: 4

INSTRUCTIONS

4 medium parsnips

1/2 white onion

4 garlic cloves

Celtic sea salt (to taste)

Ground black pepper (to taste)

Water

Bacon fat or coconut oil (for cooking)

INSTRUCTIONS

1. Heat large pan with lid over medium heat. Add 2 tablespoons bacon fat or coconut oil to hot pan.

2. Peel and mince or finely grate onion and garlic. Add to hot oiled pan and sauté until golden and aromatic, about 2 minutes.

3. Peel and slice or chop parsnips. Add to pan with 2 cups water. Increase heat to high and bring to a simmer. Cover pan loosely with lid. Cook partially covered until parsnips soften and most of the water has evaporated, about 10 minutes.

4. Pour parsnips, onions and garlic into food processor or high-speed blender. Process until thick, smooth mixture forms.

5. Transfer to serving dish and serve immediately.

Blueberry Morning Drink

Prep time: 5 minutes

INGREDIENTS

1 handful spinach

½ avocado

1 banana

½ cup blueberries

1 tbsp coconut oil

1 tsp cinnamon

1 cup water

INSTRUCTIONS

1. Slice avocado in half and remove the nut. Break the banana into small pieces.
2. Combine all ingredients except for the spinach into a blender. Blend them until pureed, then add spinach and blend until pureed.
3. Serve or chill and then serve.

Nutritional Blend

Prep time: 5 minutes

INGREDIENTS

1 handful Kale

1 banana

1 large cucumber

1 handful green beans

1 tbsp coconut oil

1 tsp cinnamon

1 cup water

INSTRUCTIONS

1. Break the banana into small pieces. De-stem the kale, skin and chop the cucumber and de-stem the green beans.
2. Combine all ingredients except for kale in a blender. Blend them until pureed, then add kale and blend until pureed.
3. Serve or chill and then serve.

Homemade Applesauce

Prep Time: 10 minutes

Cook Time: 20 minutes

Servings: 4

INGREDIENTS

2 sweet apples

2 tart apples

1/4 cup sweetener*

3/4 cup water

1/2 teaspoon ground cinnamon

1/4 teaspoon ground ginger

INSTRUCTIONS

1. Peel, core and chop apples. Add to medium pan with sweetener, water and spices. Stir to combine.

2. Cover pan with lid, and heat pan over medium heat. Cook apples about 20 minutes. Transfer to heat-safe bowl and let cool about 5 minutes.

3. Mash apples with fork or potato masher. Then chill in refrigerator.

4. Transfer chilled applesauce to lidded container. Serve chilled or room temperature.

raw honey or agave nectar

Bacon and Sweet Potato Hash

Prep Time: 10 minutes

Cook Time: 10 minutes

Servings: 2

INGREDIENTS

8 oz nitrate-free bacon (thick cut slices or whole slab)

1 medium sweet potato

1 small white onion

1 teaspoon ground cinnamon

1 teaspoon dried thyme

1 teaspoon rosemary

INSTRUCTIONS

1. Bring medium pot to boil with lightly salted water. Leave enough room in pot for sweet potato. Heat a large skillet over high heat.
2. Chop bacon into 1/2 inch pieces or cubes. Add to hot skillet and brown. Stir occasionally with wooden spoon.
3. Peel and dice sweet potato. Add to boiling water for about 4 minutes, until tender but not mushy.
4. While potatoes and bacon cook, peel and dice onion.
5. Once browned, add onion to bacon. Sauté about 1 minute, until onions are tender and a bit caramelized.
6. Drain sweet potatoes in colander and add to skillet. Sprinkle on cinnamon, thyme and rosemary. Sauté 1 - 2 minutes, until any

excess liquid is evaporated and everything is lightly caramelized and cooked through. Serve hot.

Tuna Spread

Prep Time: 5 minutes

Servings: 1

INGREDIENTS

7oz (1 can) chunk light tuna

1 avocado

1/2 small red Onion

1 carrot

1 celery stalk

1/2 Lemon

1/2 cucumber

Ground black pepper, to taste

sea salt, to taste

Paprika, to taste

INSTRUCTIONS

1. Drain tuna. Cut celery stalk in half, and preserve larger end. Peel onion. Slice avocado in half, pit and scoop out flesh into small bowl. Mash well.

2. Finely dice onion, smaller half of celery stalk, and carrot. Add to bowl, with spices to taste.

3. Add tuna to bowl, plus squeeze of lemon. Mix until combined and smooth.

4. Slice reserved half of celery stalk into sticks. Slice cucumber into 1/3 inch round.

5. Serve tuna in bowl with cucumber chips and celery sticks.

Olive Tapenade

Prep Time: 15 minutes

Servings: 2

INGREDIENTS

1 1/2 cups any combination pitted olives (Kalamata, Spanish, black, etc.) *

2 tablespoons capers

2 anchovy fillets

1 garlic clove

2 fresh basil leaves

1/2 lemon

2 tablespoons coconut oil

INSTRUCTIONS

1. Peel garlic and add to food processor or high-speed blender. Process until finely ground.

2. Rinse and drain olives, capers and anchovy fillets. Add to processor with basil, oil and squeeze of 1/2 lemon. Process until finely chopped or coarsely ground, about 1 - 2 minutes.

3. Transfer to serving dish and serve immediately.

*no pimento-stuffed olives

Quick Raw Avocado Slaw

Prep Time: 10 minutes*

Cook Time: 20 minutes

Servings: 4

INGREDIENTS

1/2 head cabbage (2 cups shredded)

1 avocado

1 carrot

Zest of 1 lemon

Juice of 1 lemon

1 tablespoon raw honey

2 tablespoons apple cider vinegar

1 teaspoon ground white pepper (or black pepper)

1 teaspoon sea salt

INSTRUCTIONS

1. Cut avocado in half and remove pit. Scoop flesh into large mixing bowl and mash with fork.
2. Remove any tough outer leaves and core from cabbage. Shred cabbage and carrot. Add to bowl with vinegar, honey, salt and pepper. Zest *then* juice lemon, and add.
3. Toss to combine.
4. Serve immediately. Or and place in refrigerator for 20 minutes and serve chilled.

Parchment Baked Salmon

Prep Time: 5 minutes

Cook Time: 20 minutes

Servings: 1

INGREDIENTS

8 oz salmon fillet (deboned, skin-on)

6 - 8 medium asparagus stalks

1/2 lemon

1 basil sprig

1 rosemary sprig

1 teaspoon coconut oil

Pinch black pepper

Pinch sea salt

Parchment paper

Kitchen twine

INSTRUCTIONS

1. Place large sheet pan on bottom rack of oven. Preheat oven to 400 degrees F. prepare parchment sheet.

2. Place salmon in middle of parchment sheet skin-side down and sprinkle with salt and pepper. Place asparagus stalks next to salmon. Cut lemon into thin slices and place over fish and asparagus. Rub herbs between palms, then lay basil and rosemary

sprig over lemon slices. Drizzle 1 teaspoon coconut oil over salmon and asparagus.

3. Gather edges of parchment up over salmon and tie tightly with kitchen twine to form sealed pouch.

4. Place pouch directly on hot baking sheet in hot oven. Bake for 20 minutes.

5. Remove from oven and carefully transfer pouch to serving plate. Carefully open pouch to release steam.

6. Serve hot.

Peppercorn Crusted Filet Mignon

Prep Time: 5 minutes

Cook Time: 5 minutes

Servings: 2

INGREDIENTS

2 (6 oz) filet mignon steaks

1 tablespoons coconut oil

1 tablespoon black peppercorns

1/2 teaspoon sea salt

1 tablespoons coconut oil

INSTRUCTIONS

1. Heat medium pan over medium-high heat and add 1 tablespoon coconut oil.
2. Place peppercorns in a plastic kitchen bag or parchment pouch and place on cutting board other counter. Crack peppercorns with heavy rolling pin or pan until broken.
3. Add cracked peppercorns to small mixing bowl with coconut oil and mix to combine.
4. Sprinkle steaks with salt , then rub with peppercorn mixture, coating evenly on both sides.
5. Place seasoned steaks in hot oiled pan and cook 2 - 4 minutes per side, for rare to medium rare. Carefully flip half way through cooking, and disturb only this once.

6. Transfer seared steaks a cutting board and let rest at least 5 minutes.
7. Serve warm with your favorite grilled veggies. Or slice with sharp knife and serve.

Seafood Paella

Prep Time: 10 minutes

Cook Time: 25 minutes

Servings: 4

INGREDIENTS

1 large head cauliflower

8 oz chorizo (or other smoked sausage)

8 oz large shrimp

12 live little neck clams

12 live mussels

4 bone-in chicken thighs

1 cup chicken stock (or seafood stock)

1 small white onion

1 teaspoon saffron

Pinch ground black pepper

Pinch sea salt

2 tablespoons coconut oil

INSTRUCTIONS

1. Heat large pan over medium heat and add coconut oil.

2. Peel and chop onion. Add to hot oiled pan and sauté until translucent, about 2 minutes.

3. Add chicken thighs and brown about 5 minutes. Turn chicken over and cook another 5 minutes.

4. Rinse and clean clams and mussels, and remove any beards with pliers. Peel and devein shrimp. Cut chorizo into 1 inch slices. Set aside.

5. Roughly chop cauliflower and add to food processor with shredding attachment, process to "rice." Or mince cauliflower with knife.

6. Add riced or minced cauliflower to chicken and sauté 2 minutes. Add chorizo, clams, mussels and shrimp. Add saffron and sauté another 2 minutes.

7. Add chicken or seafood stock and stir to combine. Increase heat to high and bring to simmer. Reduce heat to medium-high and cover. Let simmer about 5 - 7 minutes, until liquid evaporates, shrimp is opaque, and mussels and clams open. Discard any that do not open.

8. Plate and serve hot.

Garlic and Herb Escargot

Prep Time: 15 minutes

Cook Time: 15 minutes

Servings: 4

INGREDIENTS

1 lb fresh escargot (in shell)

1 /2 cup coconut oil

1 shallot

1 garlic clove

1/2 large lemon

Medium bunch fresh parsley

1/4 teaspoon ground black pepper

sea salt, to taste

INSTRUCTIONS

1. Rinse escargot under warm water. Dry shells with paper towel, then set aside.
2. Peel and mince shallot and garlic. Mince parsley. Add to small mixing bowl with coconut oil, juice of 1/2 lemon, salt and pepper. Mix until well combined.
3. With small spoon, scoop small amount of herb mixture in each shell of escargot. Fill shells until all herb mixture is used.
4. Refrigerate filled escargot shells for 5 - 10 minutes, until fat solidifies.

5. Set oven to 350 degrees F.

6. Transfer escargot to baking dish and place in oven. Cook 10 - 15 minutes, until escargot is just cooked and tender.

7. Remove from oven and serve hot. Or allow to cool slightly and serve warm.

Chicken and "Rice"

Prep Time: 10 minutes

Cook Time: 30 minutes

Servings: 4

INGREDIENTS

16 oz (1 lb) skin-on bone-in chicken

1/3 head cauliflower

4 cups chicken broth (or stock)

2 large carrots

2 large celery stalks

2 teaspoons dried thyme

3 bay leaves

1 teaspoon ground black pepper (or white pepper)

Celtic sea salt, to taste

INSTRUCTIONS

1. Heat medium pot over medium-high heat. Place chicken skin-side down in hot pot. Sear and render out fat for about 5 minutes. Turn and brown on flesh side about 5 minutes.

2. Add cauliflower to food processor with shredding attachment and process to "rice." Or mince. Set aside. Dice carrots and celery.

3. Remove chicken from hot pot and set aside. Add veggies to pot and sauté about 5 minutes.

4. Add chicken back to pot with chicken stock, spices and salt, to taste. Increase heat to high and bring to simmer. Let simmer about 15 minutes, until veggies are tender and chicken is cooked through.
5. Transfer to serving dish and serve immediately.

Bacon Baked Apples

Prep Time: 15 minutes

Cook Time: 30 minutes

Servings: 4

INGREDIENTS

6 oz nitrate-free bacon (thick slices or whole slab)

4 tart apples

4 dried apricots

2 tablespoons dried cranberries

2 tablespoons dried cherries

2 tablespoons dried raisins

1 tablespoon cinnamon

Juice of half a lemon

Zest of half a lemon

Water

INSTRUCTIONS

1. Preheat oven to 350 degrees F. Heat medium skillet over medium-high heat.

2. Chop apricots. Add dried fruit to small bowl with lemon juice. Add enough water just to cover fruit. Let fruit rehydrate for 10 minutes.

3. Dice bacon and add to hot skillet. Sauté about 5 - 8 minutes, until crisp and golden brown.

4. Slice apples in half lengthwise. Carefully core apples, scooping out seeds, stem and tough core with melon baller. Leave good-sized well in apple.
5. Arrange apples in baking dish just large enough to fit them snuggly. Pour water into bottom of baking dish, about 1/8 inch.
6. Strain fruit, reserving liquid in small bowl. Strain bacon, reserving liquid. Mix lemon zest, cinnamon and bacon with fruit.
7. Fill apple wells with fruit mixture. Press down into apple, packing slightly.
8. Pour 1 teaspoon reserved liquid and over each apple. Follow by 1 tablespoon bacon grease over all 8 apple halves.
9. Bake in preheated oven for 20 - 30 minutes, until apples are tender.
10. Serve warm. Or allow to cooled completely, and store in lidded container.

Sautéed Mongolian Beef

Prep Time: 15 minutes

Cook Time: 10 minutes

Servings: 2

INGREDIENTS

16 oz (1 lb) beef flank steak

1/4 cup arrowroot powder

2 large green onions

Coconut oil (for cooking)

Sauce

1/3 cup date butter (or raw honey or agave)

1/4 cup pure fish sauce

1/4 cup tamari (or liquid aminos or coconut aminos)

1/4 inch piece ginger

2 garlic cloves

1/2 cup water

Bacon fat or coconut oil (for cooking)

INSTRUCTIONS

1. Add arrowroot to shallow dish. Cut steak against the grain into 1/4 inch pieces. Dip each piece into arrowroot and lightly coat on both sides. Set aside for 10 minutes.

2. Heat large pan or wok over medium heat. Add about 1 cup coconut oil to hot pan.

3. Add coated beef to hot oil and cook for about 3 - 4 minutes, gently can carefully stirring constantly. Use slotted spoon to remove beef from oil and drain on paper towels. Set aside.

4. For *Sauce*, heat medium pan over medium heat. Add 1 tablespoon bacon fat or coconut oil to hot pan.

5. Peel and finely grate ginger and garlic. Add to medium pan and sauté until just golden and aromatic, about 30 seconds. Add fish sauce, tamari, date butter and water. Stir and cook until reduced and thickened, about 2 - 3 minutes.

6. Slice green onions on a diagonal into 1 inch pieces. Add to sauce with beef and sauté about 1 minute.

7. Transfer to serving dish and serve hot.

Southern Liver and Onions

Prep Time: 20 minutes*

Cook Time: 25 minutes

Servings: 4

INSTRUCTIONS

20 oz (1 1/4 lb) calves liver

2 onions (yellow or white)

4 slices nitrate-free bacon

1 lemon

2 tablespoons arrowroot powder

1/2 teaspoon Celtic sea salt

1/2 teaspoon cracked black pepper (or ground black pepper)

 Bacon fat or coconut oil (for cooking)

INSTRUCTIONS

1. *Remove thin outer membrane from liver and slice into 1/4 inch fillets. Add to glass container. Juice lemon into container and toss to coat. Cover well and refrigerate overnight.
2. Heat large cast-iron pan or skillet set over medium heat.
3. Cut bacon lengthwise into long, thin strips. Then cut in thirds crosswise and add to hot pan. Sauté bacon and let crisp, about 5 minutes. Stir occasionally. Decrease heat to medium-low.

4. Peel and thinly slice onions. Add to bacon and sauté until caramelized, about 10 minutes. Stir occasionally. Remove caramelized onions and bacon from pan and set aside.

5. Drain liver fillets in colander in sink. Rinse under running water, then pat dry.

6. In shallow dish, add arrowroot powder, salt and pepper. Mix with fork to combine.

7. Dredge liver slices in arrowroot mixture and shake off excess. Place coated liver fillets on a plate and coat remaining liver fillets.

8. Add 2 tablespoons bacon fat or coconut oil to hot pan. Add single layer of coated liver to hot oiled pan and sear for 1 minute per side. Place liver on paper towel to drain. Repeat with remaining liver.

9. Transfer liver to serving dish. Top with caramelized onions and bacon. Serve immediately .

Chicken Garlic Roast

Prep time: 10 minutes

Cook time: 25 minutes

Serves: 4

INGREDIENTS

4 pieces grass-fed chicken thighs

4 cloves garlic

4 stems rosemary

3 tbsp extra-virgin olive oil

1 lemon

¼ tsp ground black pepper

½ cup organic chicken stock

INSTRUCTIONS

1. Preheat oven to 450 degrees.
2. Strip the leaves from the rosemary and crush the garlic. Grate the lemon into zest and juice and separate the two.
3. Place chicken on a baking dish. Add garlic, rosemary, lemon zest, olive oil and ground black pepper. Toss chicken to coat thoroughly and roast (uncovered) 20 minutes.
4. After 20 minutes of roasting, add chicken broth and lemon juice. Turn over chicken.
5. Return to oven, turn oven off and let sit 5 minutes longer.

6. Remove from oven and place on serving dish, pouring pan juices over the chicken. Serve immediately or chill 20 minutes and serve.

Salmon with Berry Chutney

Prep time: 10 minutes

Cook time: 15 minutes

Serves: 4

INGREDIENTS

4 salmon filets

16 stalks of asparagus

1 cup blueberries

1 onion

1 clove garlic

1 tbsp ginger root

¼ cup apple cider vinegar

½ tsp cinnamon

INSTRUCTIONS

1. Preheat your broiler. Finely chop the onion, garlic and ginger. Prepare a stove-top pot to steam the asparagus.
2. Combine blueberry, onion, garlic, ginger, apple cider vinegar and cinnamon in a saucepan and bring to a simmer, stirring continuously. Remove from heat once it has thickened into a sauce and set aside to cool.

3. Steam the asparagus for 3-5 minutes and broil the fish for 5-7 minutes. Remove from oven.

4. Lay one piece of fish across each plate and pour the blueberry chutney over top. Lay 4 stalks of asparagus over each piece of fish and serve.

Easy Baked Chicken

Prep time: 10 minutes

Cook time: 25 minutes

Serves: 4

INGREDIENTS

4 pieces grass-fed chicken thighs

4 cloves garlic

4 stems rosemary

3 tbsp extra-virgin olive oil

1 lemon

¼ tsp ground black pepper

½ cup organic chicken stock

INSTRUCTIONS

1. Preheat oven to 450 degrees.
2. Strip the leaves from the rosemary and crush the garlic. Grate the lemon into zest and juice and separate the two.
3. Place chicken on a baking dish. Add garlic, rosemary, lemon zest, olive oil and ground black pepper. Toss chicken to coat thoroughly and roast (uncovered) 20 minutes.
4. After 20 minutes of roasting, add chicken broth and lemon juice. Turn over chicken.
5. Return to oven, turn oven off and let sit 5 minutes longer.

6. Remove from oven and place on serving dish, pouring pan juices over the chicken. Serve immediately or chill 20 minutes and serve.

Holiday Baked Ham

Prep Time: 10 minutes

Cook Time: 5 hours

Servings: 12

INGREDIENTS

1 (12 lb) bone-in ham

1 (20 oz) can organic pineapple rings (in juice)

1/2 cup date butter (or raw honey or agave)

1/2 cup whole cloves

1/2 cup water

1 lemon

1 lime

1 orange

About 12 pitted cherries (optional)

Toothpicks (optional)

INSTRUCTIONS

1. Preheat oven to 325 degrees F.
2. Drain pineapple juice into small mixing bowl. Juice lemon, lime and orange into bowl. Add sweetener and water. Mix well.
3. Place ham in roasting pan and score rind in crosshatch (diamond) pattern with knife.

4. Press cloves into rind. Place cherries on rind and secure with toothpick. Hang pineapple rings on cherries.
5. Pour pineapple juice mixture over ham and bake uncovered 4 - 5 hours, until internal temperature reaches 160 degrees F. Baste with juices about every 30 minutes.
6. Remove ham from oven. Remove toothpicks and carve. Serve hot.

Rack of Lamb with Mint Sauce

Prep Time: 5 minutes*

Cook Time: 25 minutes

Servings: 2

INGREDIENTS

1 rack of lamb with 7 - 8 ribs (about 3/4 lb)

2 tablespoons date butter (or raw honey or agave)

1 teaspoon fresh thyme

1 teaspoon fresh rosemary

1/2 teaspoon cracked black pepper (or ground black pepper)

1/2 teaspoon ground cinnamon (optional)

1 tablespoon coconut oil

Fresh Mint Sauce

1/2 cup fresh mint leaves

2 tablespoons raw honey (or agave or date butter)

1/3 cup apple cider vinegar or (coconut aminos)

INSTRUCTIONS

1. *Chop rosemary and thyme. Rub herbs, spices and salt into lamb. Cover and set aside 45 - 60 minutes.

2. Preheat oven to 475 degrees F. Coat baking dish just large enough to fit rack of lamb with coconut oil.

3. Place lamb in prepared baking dish and roast for 10 minutes. Reduce temperature to 375 degrees F and continue to cook for 10 - 15 minutes, for rare to medium-rare.

4. For *Fresh Mint Sauce*, add mint, vinegar and sweetener to food processor or high-speed blender. Process until smooth, about 1 - 2 minutes. Transfer to serving dish.

5. Remove lamb from oven and let rest about 5 minutes.

6. Cut rack of lamb into individual lamb chops and transfer to serving dish. Serve warm with *Fresh Mint Sauce*.

Bacon Wrapped Filet Mignon

Prep Time: 5 minutes

Cook Time: 20 minutes

Servings: 2

INGREDIENTS

2 (6 oz each) filet mignon steaks

2 thick slices nitrate-free bacon

Ground black pepper, to taste

Celtic sea salt, to taste

1 tablespoon coconut oil (optional)

Toothpicks

INSTRUCTIONS

1. Preheat oven to 350 degrees F. Heat medium oven-safe pan or skillet over medium heat.

2. Add bacon to hot pan. Cook and render out fat for about 5 minutes, until about halfway cooked. Remove bacon from pan and set aside, reserving bacon fat in pan. Add coconut oil to pan, if desired.

3. Wrap par-cooked bacon around steaks and secure with toothpick. Sprinkle steaks with salt and pepper to taste.

4. Add wrapped seasoned steaks to hot oiled pan and sear 2 minutes per side. Carefully flip half way through cooking.

5. Remove pan from stove and place in preheated oven. Cook about 8 - 10 minutes, until bacon is cooked through and steak is medium-rare.

6. Remove steaks from oven and transfer to cutting board. Set aside and let rest at least 2 minutes.

7. Transfer to serving dish and serve hot.

Herb Roasted Pork Tenderloin

Prep Time: 10 minutes*

Cook Time: 15 minutes

Servings: 4

INGREDIENTS

1 pork tenderloin

1 teaspoon dried rosemary

1 teaspoon dried thyme

1 teaspoon dried oregano

1 teaspoon dried basil

1 teaspoon dried marjoram (optional)

1/2 teaspoon ground black pepper

1 teaspoon Celtic sea salt

Apricot Sauce

1 cup dried apricots

2/3 cup water

1 teaspoon apple cider vinegar

INSTRUCTIONS

1. Preheat oven to 425 degrees F. Heat small pan over medium heat.
2. Rub tenderloin with salt and spices, then press into meat so it adheres. Place on sheet pan, or wire rack over sheet pan.

3. Roast for 10 - 15 minutes, until just cooked through and no pink remains. Remove pork from oven and let rest 10 minutes.

4. For *Apricot Sauce*, add dried apricots, water and vinegar to food processor or high-speed blender. Process until smooth, about 1 - 2 minutes.

5. Add *Apricot Sauce* to hot pan and reduce until slightly thickened. Stir well and do not let burn. Remove from heat.

6. Slice pork and transfer to serving dish. Top pork with *Apricot Sauce* and serve warm.

Pan Seared Duck

Prep Time: 10 minutes

Cook Time: 15 minutes

Servings: 2

INGREDIENTS

2 (8 oz each) boneless duck breast halves (with skin and fat)

1 teaspoon raw honey

2 teaspoons dried thyme

1 sprig rosemary

1/2 teaspoon ground black pepper

1 teaspoons Celtic sea salt

INSTRUCTIONS

1. Heat medium pan or skillet over medium-high heat.
2. Rinse duck breast and pat dry with paper towel.
3. Rub rosemary spring between palms, then remove needles from stem and chop. Rub rosemary, thyme, salt and pepper into both sides of duck breasts.
4. Drizzle honey over fatty side of duck breast, then place in hot oiled pan, skin and fat side down. Let brown undisturbed for 5 minutes. Turn duck over with tongs and cook until desired doneness, 5 - 10 minutes for medium to well done.
5. Transfer duck breasts to cutting board and cover with aluminum foil. Set aside to rest 5 minutes.

6. Cut each duck breast in 1/2 inch diagonal slices. Transfer to serving dish and serve warm.

Apple Venison Roast

Prep Time: 10 minutes

Cook Time: 7 hours

Servings: 6

INGREDIENTS

3 lbs boneless venison roast (deer roast)

1/2 cup apple juice

2 firm apples

1 onion (yellow or white)

4 cloves garlic

1 teaspoon Celtic sea salt

INSTRUCTIONS

1. Sprinkle venison with salt and add to slow cooker.
2. Peel garlic and smash. Peel onion and quarter. Peel apples, then cut in half and core. Add to slow cooker with apple juice.
3. Cover slow cooker with lid. Turn on to low and cook 6 - 8 hours, until meat is tender.
4. Turn off slow cooker and carefully remove lid. Remove roast and slice.
5. Transfer to serving dish and serve hot with apples and onions, if preferred.

Kelp Noodle Chicken Soup

Prep Time: 10 minutes

Cook Time: 45 minutes

Servings: 4

INGREDIENTS

3 package (12 oz) kelp noodles

32 oz (2 lbs) skin-on bone-in chicken

4 cups chicken broth (or stock)

2 large carrots

2 large celery stalks

2 teaspoons dried thyme

3 bay leaves

1 teaspoon ground black pepper (or white pepper)

Celtic sea salt, to taste

Water

INSTRUCTIONS

1. Heat medium pot over medium heat. Place chicken skin-side down in hot pot. Brown for about 5 minutes on each side. Remove browned chicken and set aside.

2. Dice carrots and celery. Add veggies to pot and sauté about 5 minutes.

3. Rinse and drain kelp noodles. Add to pot with chicken, chicken stock, spices and salt, to taste. Bring to simmer, then reduce heat to low.

4. Let simmer about 30 minutes, until veggies are tender and chicken is cooked through.

5. Transfer to serving dish and serve immediately.

Butternut Squash Soup

Prep Time: 10 minutes

Cook Time: 1 hour

Servings: 4

INGREDIENTS

1 medium-large butternut squash (about 2 cups diced)

2 cups chicken stock (or veggie stock)

1/2 cup coconut milk (optional)

1/2 onion (white, yellow or sweet)

1/2 large carrot

1/2 celery stalk

1 cinnamon stick

Ground black pepper, to taste

Celtic sea salt, to taste

2 tablespoons coconut oil (or bacon fat)

2 tablespoons bacon fat (or coconut oil)

INSTRUCTIONS

1. Heat oven to 375 degrees F. Heat medium cast iron pan over medium-high heat. Add bacon fat to hot oiled pan.

2. Peel squash and remove seeds. Dice and add to hot oiled pan with salt and pepper, to taste. Sauté until golden, about 3 - 4 minutes. Place pan in oven and roast until browned on all sides, about 15 minutes.

3. Heat medium pot over medium-low heat. Add coconut oil to hot pot.

4. Peel and dice onion, celery and carrot. Add to hot oiled pot with cinnamon stick, salt and pepper to taste. Sauté until soft but not browned, about 10 minutes.

5. Remove squash from oven and let cool slightly. Add food processor or high-speed blender and process until puréed.

6. Add chicken broth to pot. Increase heat to medium and bring to boil. Simmer about 5 minutes.

7. Stir in squash purée and simmer about 10 minutes. Discard cinnamon stick.

8. Add mixture to food processor or high-speed blender and purée until smooth. Or blend with immerse or stick blender until smooth.

9. Transfer mixture back to hot pot and stir in coconut milk (optional). Transfer to serving dish.

10. Sprinkle with cracked black pepper. Serve hot.

New England Clam Chowder

Prep Time: 10 minutes

Cook Time: 40 minutes

Servings: 4

INGREDIENTS

24 - 36 medium live littleneck clams (or other clam varieties)

2 cans (14 oz) full-fat coconut milk

3 - 4 cups clam juice (or fish stock or chicken stock)

4 slices nitrate-free bacon

4 medium parsnips

1 small onion

1 garlic clove

1 tablespoon tapioca flour (or arrow root powder)

1 1/2 teaspoons ground white black pepper (or black pepper)

1 teaspoon Celtic sea salt

Small bunch fresh parsley (for garnish)

Water

INSTRUCTIONS

1. Have fishmonger shuck clams. Or carefully shuck clams yourself. Reserve clam juice. Chop clams, if desired, and add to reserved clam juice. Set aside in refrigerator.

2. Heat medium pot over medium-high heat. Chop bacon and add to hot pot. Sauté until crisp, about 5 - 7 minutes. Stir occasionally.

3. Peel and roughly chop onion. Peel garlic. Add to food processor and pulse until finely chopped, about 1 minute. Or mince. Chop parsnips.

4. Drain bacon on paper towels. Set aside. Reserve bacon fat in hot pot.

5. Add onion, garlic, tapioca salt and pepper to hot oiled pot. Sauté until fragrant, about 2 minutes.

6. Add parsnips. Stir in coconut milk and 2 - 3 cups clam juice. Reduce heat to low and simmer for 20 minutes.

7. Remove clams in their juice from refrigerator and add to pot. Stir in remaining clam juice, if desired. Bring to simmer, then cook another 5 minutes.

8. Transfer to serving dishes. Chop parsley and sprinkle over dish with chopped bacon.

9. Serve immediately.

Spinach Artichoke Soup

Prep Time: 5 minutes

Cook Time: 30 minutes

Servings: 4

INGREDIENTS

2 cups vegetable broth (or chicken broth)

1 can (13.5 oz) full-fat coconut milk

4 cups spinach leaves

1 1/2 cups artichoke hearts (canned or jarred, drained)

1/2 small onion (yellow or white)

1 garlic clove

1 teaspoon ground white pepper (or ground black pepper)

2 teaspoons Celtic sea salt

1 tablespoon bacon fat (or coconut oil)

INSTRUCTIONS

1. Heat medium pot over medium heat. Add fat to hot pot.
2. Peel and thinly slice onion. Peel and finely grate or mince garlic. Add to hot oiled pot and sauté until tender and translucent, about 5 minutes.
3. Fill pot with spinach and stir to wilt. Continue until all spinach is added. Stir in salt and pepper.
4. Chop artichoke hearts and add to pot with veggie broth and coconut milk. Stir to combine.

5. Bring to simmer and heat through, about 8 - 10 minutes.

6. Transfer to serving dish and serve hot.

Cream of Mushroom Soup

Prep Time: 5 minutes

Cook Time: 30 minutes

Servings: 4

INGREDIENTS

3 cups vegetable broth (or chicken broth)

1 can (13.5 oz) full-fat coconut milk

4 cups mushrooms (white, baby bella, etc.)

1/2 onion (yellow or white)

1 garlic clove

1 teaspoon ground white pepper (or ground black pepper)

2 teaspoons Celtic sea salt

2 tablespoons bacon fat (or coconut oil)

INSTRUCTIONS

1. Heat large pot over medium-high heat. Add 1 tablespoon fat to hot pot.
2. Slice 1 cup mushrooms and add to pot. Sauté until lightly browned and tender, about 5 minutes. Remove from pot and set aside.
3. Add remaining fat to hot pot. Reduce heat to medium.
4. Peel and chop onions and garlic. Add to hot oiled pot and sauté until fragrant and lightly browned, about 5 minutes.
5. Add whole mushrooms to pot and sauté until lightly browned and tender, about 8 - 10 minutes.

6. Transfer mushrooms, onion and garlic to food processor or high-speed blender with vegetable broth, coconut milk, salt and pepper. Process until smooth, about 1 - 2 minutes.
7. Or add vegetable broth, coconut milk, salt and pepper to pot and purée with immersion blender.
8. Heat pot over medium heat. Add reserved sliced mushrooms to pot and stir to combine.
9. Bring to simmer and heat through, about 8 - 10 minutes.
10. Transfer to serving dish and serve hot.

Smoked Salmon Avocado Salad

Prep Time: 10 minutes

Servings: 1

INGREDIENTS

Salad

2 cups soft lettuce leaves (looseleaf or butterhead varieties)

1/2 cup watercress or dandelion leaves (optional)

2 oz smoked salmon

1/2 avocado

1 sprig fresh dill

1 tablespoon caviar (optional)

Avocado Cream Dressing

1/2 avocado

1 sprig fresh dill

1 tablespoon lemon juice

1/2 teaspoon ground black pepper

1/2 teaspoon Celtic sea salt

1/2 coconut

Water

INSTRUCTIONS

1. For *Salad*, rinse, dry and plate lettuce and watercress or dandelion leaves (optional). Cut avocado in half and remover pit. Dice or

slice avocado flesh in peel, then scoop onto greens. Lay smoked salmon over greens.

2. For *Avocado Cream Dressing*, remove coconut flesh from peel and add to food processor or high-speed blender with enough water to reach desired consistency. Process until smooth and creamy, about 1 - 2 minutes. Strain mixture through nut milk bag and place back into blender.

3. Scoop remaining avocado flesh into blender. Add lemon juice, 1 sprig dill, salt and pepper and process until well combined and smooth, about 1 minute.

4. Drizzle *Avocado Cream Dressing* over salad. Mince remaining dill and sprinkle over salad. Dollop caviar over salad (optional).

5. Serve immediately.

Avocado Persimmon Salad

Prep Time: 10 minutes*

Servings: 2

INGREDIENTS

2 persimmons

1 avocado

1 medium cucumber

1/2 sweet onion

2 tablespoons raw oil (coconut, olive, etc.)

2 tablespoon lemon juice (or lime juice or raw apple cider vinegar)

1/2 teaspoon cracked or ground black pepper

1/4 teaspoon Celtic sea salt

INSTRUCTIONS

1. Peel and seed cucumber if preferred, then dice. Peel persimmons if preferred, then chop. Peel sweet onions and cut in half. Thinly slice. Add to medium mixing bowl.
2. Cut avocado in half and remove pit. Dice peel in flesh and scoop into bowl.
3. Add oil, lemon juice, salt and pepper. Toss to coat evenly
4. Transfer to serving dishes and serve immediately.
5. *Or refrigerate for 20 minutes and serve chilled.

Kelp Noodle Salad

Prep Time: 5 minutes

Cook Time: 5 minutes

Servings: 2

INGREDIENTS

1 package (12 oz) kelp noodles

1/2 lemon

1 small cucumber

1 large carrot

Small bunch cilantro

2 large basil leaves

Orange Avocado Dressing

1 avocado

1 large orange

1/2 lemon

5 large basil leaves

1/4 teaspoon ground black pepper

Large bunch cilantro

INSTRUCTIONS

1. Rinse and drain kelp noodles. Add to medium bowl and soak 5 minutes in warm water and juice of 1/2 lemon. Or bring medium

pot of water with juice of 1/2 lemon to a boil and cook kelp noodles for 5 minutes, if softer texture preferred.

2. Peel, seed and cut cucumber in half width-wise. Cut bell pepper in half, then remove stem, seeds and veins. Use vegetable peeler or grater to make long, thin slices of carrot. Thinly slice cucumber lengthwise.

3. Add veggies and drained kelp noodles to medium mixing bowl.

4. For *Orange Avocado Dressing*, add basil and cilantro leaves to food processor or bullet blender with juice of orange and process to break down leaves. Slice avocado in half and remove pit. Scoop flesh into processor with juice of 1/2 lemon and black pepper. Process until thick and until creamy.

5. Pour *Orange Avocado Dressing* over sliced veggies and kelp noodles. Toss to coat.

6. Serve immediately. Or refrigerate for 20 minutes and serve chilled.

Salmon & Veggie Breakfast Salad

Prep Time: 10 minutes

Cook Time: 10 minutes

Servings: 1

INGREDIENTS

Salad:

1 medium salmon fillet (or 2 oz smoked salmon, do not cook)

1 carrot

1/2 cucumber

8 asparagus stalks

1 cup cabbage

1/2 lemon

Dressing:

1 avocado

2 tablespoons coconut oil

1/2 lemon

1 small clove garlic

1 tablespoon fresh parsley

1 tablespoon fresh dill

Pinch sea salt

Pinch ground black pepper

INSTRUCTIONS

1. Bring small pot to boil with salted water. Heat small skillet over medium-high heat and lightly coat with coconut oil.

2. Parboil asparagus spears in boiling water for about 2 minutes. Then drain and shock in ice bath.

3. Lay salmon fillet skin-side down in hot oiled skillet. Cook about 3 minutes on each side. Season to taste, then squeeze lemon juice over fillet.

4. Shred or grate cabbage, carrot and cucumber. Drain cucumber in paper towel. Dry asparagus in paper towel and slice into 2 inch pieces. Toss veggies together.

5. Peel garlic and add all **Dressing** ingredients with squeeze of lemon, salt and pepper to taste to food processor or bullet blender. Process until smooth.

6. Plate shredded veggies. Remove salmon fillet and flake off meat over shredded veggies. Or lay smoked salmon slices over veggies.

7. Drizzle salad with avocado **Dressing**. Squeeze a little more lemon juice over salad. Serve immediately.

Chapter 6 - Conclusion

Eating healthy is the best way to keep IBS in control. Eating nutritious meals does not mean depriving yourself of delicious and indulgent foods. It does not mean limiting yourself to tasteless, flavorless, boring food. All it takes are knowing what foods and substances to stay away from and a little creativity in coming up with and preparing "IBS-friendly."

The best way to ensure that the food you eat is IBS-friendly is to cook it yourself. If you're having trouble deciding, here are recipes that you can follow to make a meal both nutritious and delicious. Some traditional recipes only need to substitute high FODMAP foods with low ones but the taste, flavor, and nutrient contents remain the same.

www.ingramcontent.com/pod-product-compliance
Lightning Source LLC
Chambersburg PA
CBHW051219170526
45166CB00005B/1961